CELLULITE REDUCTION TREATMENTS FOR BEGINNERS

Effective Home Remedies And Professional Techniques For Smooth Skin And Natural Wellness

DR SAWYER DIEGO

DISCLAMER

Nothing in this book should be interpreted as medical advice; it is meant exclusively for educational reasons. Regarding their specific health issues and treatment options, readers are urged to speak with licensed healthcare professionals. The publisher and author disclaim all liability for any errors or omissions in the material provided, as well as for any negative effects that may arise from using or abusing the information. Although every attempt has been taken to guarantee that the material in this book is correct as of the date of publishing, new research may have superseded some of the content because medical knowledge is always changing. It is recommended that readers confirm the most recent medical recommendations and guidelines. The reader of this book undertakes to release the author and publisher from any claims or liabilities resulting from the use of this information, and understands and accepts the inherent risks connected with healthcare decisions.

TABLE OF CONTENTS

ABOUT THE BOOK

Debunking common myths, this book clarifies misconceptions surrounding cellulite, shedding light on its physiological basis and why it tends to manifest in specific body areas. Cellulite, a common cosmetic concern, is thoroughly explored to provide a comprehensive understanding of its nature and formation. Cellulite Reduction Treatments for Beginners is an essential guide that aims to demystify the complexities surrounding cellulite and empower readers with effective strategies for its reduction.

The focus of the book is on developing healthy lifestyle habits; it emphasizes how important it is to have a balanced diet, exercise regularly, drink enough water, manage stress, and get enough sleep to fight cellulite.

By incorporating these practices, readers will have the fundamental knowledge they need to attain holistic wellness and treat cellulite from the inside out.

This book walks readers through a variety of cellulite reduction treatments, beginning with topical ones. It goes into great detail about the effectiveness of creams and lotions, clarifies important ingredients, and offers advice on the best ways to apply them. It also guides how to choose products that work best for them and how to combine complementary techniques to achieve even better results.

Another important component of cellulite reduction is massage therapy. This book examines various massage techniques and emphasizes how they improve blood circulation and skin texture. It provides practical advice on how to use massage therapy to reduce visible cellulite, ranging from do-it-yourself techniques to professional services.

Physical therapy and exercise are also essential elements. While alternative therapies such as radiofrequency treatments and Endermologie offer readers more treatment options, targeted exercises, cardiovascular workouts, and strength training regimens are designed to reduce the appearance of cellulite.

Diving deeper into holistic approaches, the book covers dietary supplements and how they support skin health; readers learn about important vitamins, minerals, and herbal supplements; safety is emphasized, and healthcare practitioners should be consulted for specific recommendations.

For those who are thinking about going further, medical procedures like liposuction, mesotherapy, and laser therapy are covered in great detail, along with safety precautions and expectations for the course of treatment, so that you can make an educated decision and get the best results possible.

Hydration, detoxification, herbal remedies, and dietary adjustments are investigated to complement lifestyle changes and preserve long-term effects; natural remedies and do-it-yourself therapies are highlighted for their accessibility and effectiveness in cellulite reduction.

To empower readers to take charge of their cellulite reduction journey with confidence, "Cellulite Reduction Treatments for Beginners" concludes with strategies for maintaining results and preventing cellulite recurrence. It emphasizes consistency in treatment, progress monitoring, and lifestyle adjustments for sustained improvement.

To ensure that readers are well-informed on safety, financial considerations, managing treatment side effects, and optimizing their lifestyle for continued cellulite improvement, typical concerns and frequently asked questions are thoroughly covered throughout the book.

CHAPTER ONE
CELLULITE REDUCTION TREATMENTS OVERVIEW
KNOWING WHAT CELLULITE IS AND WHY IT OCCURS

Understanding cellulite entails realizing that it's not a medical condition but rather a normal physiological process influenced by genetics, diet, lifestyle, and hormonal changes. Cellulite is a common cosmetic concern that is characterized by dimpled, lumpy skin, usually on the thighs, buttocks, and abdomen. It occurs when fat deposits push through the connective tissue beneath the skin, creating a bumpy appearance. This phenomenon is more common in women due to differences in fat distribution, connective tissue structure, and hormonal factors.

Cellulite is a result of fat cells expanding and pushing against the skin's connective tissue; these factors, along with age and lifestyle choices, all contribute to the formation of cellulite.

Despite popular belief, cellulite is not exclusively associated with body weight; hormonal fluctuations or genetic predispositions can also cause cellulite formation in lean individuals. Knowledge of these underlying mechanisms aids in the selection of appropriate treatments that address the underlying causes of cellulite formation.

To effectively address cellulite, a holistic approach combining targeted treatments with healthy lifestyle habits is necessary. These habits include eating a balanced diet high in fruits, vegetables, and lean proteins, drinking plenty of water, and exercising regularly. These lifestyle changes not only support overall health but also help to reduce the appearance of cellulite by improving skin elasticity, circulation, and fat metabolism. People can take proactive measures to achieve smoother, firmer skin by being aware of the factors that contribute to cellulite formation and embracing healthy habits.

COMMON FALSE BELIEFS AND MYTHS REGARDING CELLULITE

There are a lot of myths and misconceptions surrounding cellulite, which can lead to misconceptions about its causes and treatments. For example, it's a common misconception that cellulite is only found in overweight people. In reality, cellulite can affect people of all body types due to factors other than weight, like hormone fluctuations and genetics. Another common misconception is that cellulite is permanent or untreatable. While it can be difficult to eliminate, there are treatments and lifestyle changes that can significantly reduce its visibility.

Another common misconception is that cellulite can only be removed by topical creams. Although some creams can temporarily improve skin texture, long-term reduction necessitates a multifaceted approach including targeted treatments, exercise, and dietary modifications. Cellulite formation is more complex, involving factors such as hormones, collagen structure, and fat distribution. Addressing these underlying causes is crucial for effective cellulite reduction.

Cellulite myths and realities must be understood for people to make well-informed decisions regarding available treatments. By clearing up myths and emphasizing evidence-based methods, people can more confidently navigate the wide range of cellulite treatments available. Accurate information combined with doable tactics encourages people to take proactive measures toward having smoother, healthier-looking skin.

THE VALUE OF HEALTHFUL LIVING PRACTICES

A balanced diet that includes lots of fresh fruits, vegetables, whole grains, and lean proteins provides essential nutrients that support skin health and overall well-being. Hydration is also important because it supports detoxification processes and helps to maintain skin elasticity. Regular exercise, such as strength training and cardiovascular activities, improves circulation, tones muscles, and promotes fat metabolism, which helps to reduce the appearance of cellulite and promote smoother skin texture.

Stress management is also important because stress can cause hormonal imbalances, which in turn can lead to the formation of cellulite. Stress management techniques, such as yoga, meditation, or regular relaxation exercises, can help reduce stress and support overall skin health. Reducing alcohol and cigarette consumption is also important because these substances can impair circulation and collagen production, which can exacerbate the appearance of cellulite. Adequate sleep is another important component because it enables the body to repair and regenerate, promoting skin renewal and elasticity.

Eating well, exercising, managing stress, getting enough sleep, and adopting a holistic approach that includes nutrition, exercise, stress management, and adequate rest empowers people to address cellulite from multiple angles and achieve smoother, firmer skin.

By prioritizing healthy lifestyle habits, individuals not only improve their overall well-being but also the efficacy of cellulite reduction treatments.

HOW YOU CAN BENEFIT FROM THIS BOOK

As a thorough guide to cellulite reduction, this book dispels common misconceptions and highlights effective treatments to provide readers with the knowledge they need to navigate the terrain of cellulite reduction. It offers clear explanations of what cellulite is, its causes, and the various myths surrounding it, empowering readers with accurate information to make informed decisions.

A valuable resource for anyone looking to improve the appearance of their skin and their general health through sustainable lifestyle changes and targeted treatments, the book emphasizes the importance of adopting healthy lifestyle habits and offers helpful advice on nutrition, exercise, stress management, and skincare routines that support cellulite reduction efforts.

It outlines realistic expectations and offers practical advice, guiding readers on a journey towards achieving smoother, firmer skin and boosting self-confidence.

Whether you're new to cellulite treatments or looking for advanced strategies, this book offers insights and guidance that can be tailored to individual needs and preferences. By understanding the principles of cellulite formation and implementing evidence-based solutions, readers can start on a path toward achieving their desired skin texture and appearance.

WHAT TO ANTICIPATE FROM TREATMENTS AIMED AT REDUCING CELLULITE

Many techniques are used in cellulite reduction treatments; these include topical creams, massages, and advanced medical procedures. The goal of each treatment is to target a different aspect of cellulite, such as fat deposits, collagen structure, and skin elasticity. Topical treatments, on the other hand, often involve the use of ingredients like caffeine or retinol, which temporarily improve skin texture and circulation. Although these creams can be beneficial in the short term, the best results usually come from consistent use combined with other lifestyle modifications.

Incorporate massage and dry brushing techniques into your everyday skincare routine to improve overall skin health and support other cellulite reduction strategies. For more focused results, medical treatments like radiofrequency, laser therapy, or ultrasound may be suggested to break down fat cells, stimulate collagen production, and tighten skin. Massages and dry brushing techniques are popular non-invasive treatments that aim to stimulate circulation and lymphatic drainage, helping to reduce fluid retention and improve skin tone.

A person can customize a cellulite reduction plan that targets their specific concerns and goals by learning about the range of options available and consulting with skincare professionals.

CHAPTER TWO
FUNDAMENTALS OF CELLULITE
CELLULITE: DEFINITION AND CAUSES

When fat deposits push through the connective tissue beneath the skin, a visibly uneven surface is created. This condition is commonly found on the thighs, buttocks, and abdomen. Women are more likely than men to have cellulite because of variations in fat distribution, connective tissue structure, and hormonal factors. Cellulite is not always an indication of obesity; people who are healthy weight can also have it.

Several factors contribute to cellulite formation: genetics, where specific genes predispose individuals to the formation of cellulite; hormonal factors, especially estrogen, which affects the structure of connective tissue and fat accumulation; lifestyle factors, including diet, lack of exercise, and smoking, which increase fat deposition and weaken connective tissue; and age-related changes in skin elasticity and collagen, which over time make cellulite more noticeable.

By addressing underlying factors like genetics, hormonal balance, lifestyle choices, and the effects of aging, individuals can better manage and reduce the appearance of cellulite through targeted treatments and lifestyle modifications. Knowing the definition and causes of cellulite is essential for selecting effective treatment strategies.

DIFFERENT CELLULITE TYPES

Depending on the appearance and severity of the condition, cellulite can take many different forms. The most common types are hard cellulite, which feels rigid and is typically found in younger people whose skin is less elastic; soft cellulite, which is more jiggly and is often found in older people whose skin, is looser; and edematous cellulite, which is defined by fluid retention and frequently accompanied by swelling and discomfort.

Treatment for each type of cellulite is different, and only a customized approach will work. For example, radiofrequency treatments or laser therapy may be beneficial for hard cellulite, while lymphatic drainage massage or topical caffeine creams may be more effective for soft cellulite. Finally, lifestyle modifications such as dietary changes and increased physical activity may be necessary for edematous cellulite to reduce fluid retention.

By identifying the specific characteristics and underlying factors contributing to the appearance of cellulite, people can take proactive steps toward achieving smoother skin and improved body confidence. Knowledge of the various types of cellulite aids both individuals and practitioners in selecting the most suitable treatment plan.

FACTORS AFFECTING THE DEVELOPMENT OF CELLULITE

Genetics plays a major role in the formation of cellulite, as certain genes can affect how fat is stored and distributed as well as the strength and elasticity of connective tissue. Hormonal factors, particularly estrogen, influence fat distribution and connective tissue composition, making women more prone to cellulite than men. Age-related changes in skin structure are another factor that contributes to the formation of cellulite.

Exercise and dietary habits can also have an impact on the development of cellulite. Diets heavy in fats, carbohydrates, and salts can exacerbate the appearance of cellulite by increasing fat deposition and fluid retention. Inactivity can cause poor circulation and decreased muscle tone, which in turn can accelerate the development of cellulite. Smoking and excessive alcohol use can also weaken the collagen and elastin fibers in the skin, making cellulite more visible.

Cellulite's visible appearance is a result of age-related changes in collagen production and skin elasticity. As skin becomes less resilient and firm, underlying fat deposits become more noticeable, giving the appearance of dimples. Knowledge of these contributing factors enables people to make well-informed decisions regarding lifestyle changes and treatments to effectively manage and reduce cellulite.

COMPREHENDING THE STRUCTURE AND APPEARANCE OF CELLULITE

The structure and composition of the skin, specifically the thickness of the dermis and the configuration of connective tissue fibers, are factors that affect cellulite. The dermis is thinner and the connective tissue forms a pattern resembling honeycomb in areas where cellulite is present, which allows fat cells to protrude through and give the skin's surface a dimpled appearance.

Skin varies in thickness throughout the body; thinner skin on regions such as the thighs and buttocks is more prone to cellulite because it shows underlying fat deposits and connective tissue structure. The skin is supported and elasticated by collagen and elastin fibers in the dermis; these fibers weaken with age or hormonal changes, making the skin less able to maintain a smooth surface, which in turn contributes to the development of cellulite.

Increasing skin elasticity, boosting collagen production, and encouraging healthy circulation are some of the ways that effective cellulite treatments address the root causes of the condition. People who are aware of how the structure of their skin affects the appearance of cellulite can select treatments that best suit their needs and maximize outcomes.

WHY CERTAIN PARTS OF THE BODY ARE MORE PRONE TO CELLULITE

The thighs, buttocks, and abdomen are common sites for cellulite formation in women, where fat cells are larger and more likely to protrude through weakened connective tissue; these areas also have thinner skin and less supportive collagen and elastin fibers, making cellulite more visible. These differences in fat distribution, connective tissue structure, and hormonal influences all contribute to the tendency for cellulite to be more prevalent in specific areas of the body.

Cellulite is more common in women than in men because of hormonal differences that impact the body's distribution and storage of fat. Specifically, estrogen increases fat accumulation in the thighs and buttocks, which is where cellulite typically forms. Hormonal factors, in particular, estrogen, play a significant role in the development of cellulite by influencing fat distribution and connective tissue composition.

Where cellulite is more likely to develop depends on genetic predisposition as well. Some genes influence the strength of connective tissue and the distribution of fat cells, making certain people more prone to cellulite formation in particular areas.

Lifestyle factors like diet, exercise routines, and smoking can aggravate cellulite by causing more fat to be deposited and weakening the structure of the skin.

Individuals can effectively target treatment strategies by knowing why particular areas of the body are more prone to cellulite. By addressing underlying factors like genetic predisposition, hormonal influences, and lifestyle choices, individuals can take proactive measures to improve skin texture and appearance while also reducing cellulite.

CHAPTER THREE

MODIFICATIONS TO YOUR LIFESTYLE TO REDUCE CELLULITE

THE SIGNIFICANCE OF NUTRITION AND DIET

A diet high in fresh fruits, vegetables, lean proteins, and whole grains provides essential nutrients that support skin elasticity and reduce inflammation. Avoiding processed foods high in sugar and unhealthy fats helps prevent weight gain, which can exacerbate cellulite. Including foods rich in antioxidants, like berries and leafy greens, helps combat free radicals that contribute to skin aging and cellulite formation. Diet plays a crucial role in managing cellulite by affecting fat storage, metabolism, and overall skin health.

Drinking plenty of water throughout the day helps flush out toxins and keeps skin cells hydrated and plump. Herbal teas and infused water can add variety while providing additional hydration benefits.

Maintaining skin elasticity and reducing the appearance of cellulite also depend on proper hydration.

SAFE PHYSICAL ACTIVITY AND EXERCISE

Frequent exercise not only helps reduce body fat overall but also tones muscles, which can improve the appearance of cellulite. Building muscle and boosting metabolism can be achieved by combining strength training exercises like squats and lunges with cardiovascular exercises like running or cycling. Targeting cellulite-prone areas like the thighs and buttocks with targeted exercises can firm and tighten the skin.

Find enjoyable activities and realistic goals to help maintain motivation and achieve long-term results. HIIT, or high-intensity interval training, can also help burn fat and improve circulation, which aids in the reduction of cellulite. Consistency is key.

HYDRATION AND ITS FUNCTION IN REDUCING CELLULITE

Water helps flush out toxins that can lead to the formation of cellulite; hydrated skin looks smoother and more supple, which reduces the dimpled appearance of cellulite. Hydration plays a critical role in reducing cellulite by improving skin elasticity and texture.

Apart from water, you may boost your hydration levels by including vegetables like celery, cucumbers, and watermelon in your diet. You can also reduce cellulite by avoiding excessive alcohol and caffeinated drink use, which are dehydrating drinks.

TECHNIQUES FOR STRESS MANAGEMENT

Chronic stress raises cortisol levels, which encourages the body to store fat. Reducing stress through deep breathing exercises, yoga, meditation, or other relaxation techniques can help lower cortisol levels and enhance general well-being. Hobbies, outdoor activities, and spending time with loved ones can also help reduce stress and support mental health.

Stress has a physiological influence on the body, including cellulite, which may be lessened by prioritizing self-care and making time for relaxation. Additionally, practicing mindfulness and maintaining a regular sleep schedule can help manage stress even more and improve general health.

THE VALUE OF REST AND RECUPERATION

The body repairs damaged tissues and balances hormone levels during sleep, including those involved in metabolism and fat storage. Poor sleep quality can disrupt these processes and contribute to weight gain and the formation of cellulite. Getting enough sleep is necessary for cellular repair and regeneration, which is essential for maintaining healthy skin and reducing cellulite.

Prioritizing sleep as part of a healthy lifestyle can support overall well-being and enhance efforts to reduce cellulite. Creating a sleep-friendly environment and establishing a bedtime routine can improve the quality and duration of sleep. Avoiding electronic devices before bedtime and practicing relaxation techniques like reading or gentle stretching can promote relaxation and prepare the body for restorative sleep.

CHAPTER FOUR

TOPICAL CELLULITE TREATMENTS

A SYNOPSIS OF TOPICAL LOTIONS AND CREAMS

Because they are non-invasive and simple to use, topical creams and lotions are a popular choice for decreasing cellulite. These products usually contain active ingredients that work to improve skin texture and reduce the appearance of cellulite. Common ingredients in these creams include caffeine, retinol, and antioxidants like vitamin C and E. Retinol stimulates the production of collagen, which improves skin elasticity. Antioxidants shield the skin from damage caused by free radicals, supporting overall skin health.

Applying topical creams and lotions directly to the afflicted areas, typically twice a day as part of a regular skincare regimen, is the key to achieving the best results. You should massage the product into the skin with upward strokes to stimulate circulation and promote absorption. These creams have the potential to improve skin firmness and smoothness over time, reducing the appearance of cellulite, but individual outcomes may differ.

RECOGNIZING THE COMPONENTS OF CELLULITE CREAMS

Retinol, a vitamin A derivative, stimulates the production of collagen and improves skin texture over time. Other ingredients like peptides help to firm and plump the skin, reducing the dimpled appearance of cellulite. One common ingredient found in cellulite creams is caffeine, which is known for its ability to increase blood flow and temporarily reduce the appearance of cellulite by tightening the skin.

The role of each ingredient can help you choose a product that aligns with your skincare goals and preferences. When choosing a cellulite cream, it's important to carefully read the ingredient list. Look for clinically proven ingredients like caffeine, retinol, and peptides, which have shown efficacy in reducing cellulite. Avoid products with potentially irritating ingredients like artificial fragrances and dyes, especially if you have sensitive skin.

APPLICATION STRATEGIES FOR OPTIMAL OUTCOMES

The key to getting the most out of cellulite creams is to apply them correctly. To begin, wash and dry your skin before applying the cream. Next, take a small amount of the product and gently massage it into your skin in upward strokes, concentrating on areas that are prone to cellulite, like your abdomen, thighs, and buttocks.

This will help to improve overall results by improving absorption, stimulating circulation, and improving overall results.

A healthy diet and regular exercise can further enhance the effects of topical treatments for cellulite reduction. Consistency is key, so apply the cellulite cream twice a day, preferably in the morning and evening, and allow the product to absorb fully before dressing to prevent staining or transfer. Results may vary depending on individual skin types and conditions, but over time, you may notice improvements in skin firmness and texture.

HOW TO SELECT THE APPROPRIATE PRODUCT

To ensure that the cellulite cream you choose is both effective and compatible with your skin type, take into account several factors. First, determine the exact skincare concerns and goals you have. Next, look for products that contain ingredients that have been clinically proven to work, such as antioxidants, retinol, and caffeine. These ingredients work to target cellulite by promoting collagen production, improving circulation, and shielding the skin from free radical damage.

Seek certifications or endorsements from dermatologists or skincare experts to verify the product's claims. Take into account your skin type and any sensitivity you may have to specific ingredients. If you have sensitive skin, go for fragrance-free and hypoallergenic options. Finally, choose products with a pleasant texture and easy application to ensure consistency in your skincare routine.

COMBINING OTHER APPROACHES WITH TOPICAL TREATMENTS

Incorporating regular exercise, such as cardio and strength training, helps to improve circulation and tone muscles, which reduces the appearance of cellulite. Maintaining a balanced diet rich in fruits, vegetables, and lean proteins supports overall skin health and collagen production. Although topical treatments can be effective on their own, combining them with other methods can enhance results in reducing cellulite.

Achieving smoother, firmer skin and effectively reducing the appearance of cellulite can be achieved by integrating multiple approaches. Drinking plenty of water and staying hydrated supports skin elasticity and detoxification processes. Professional treatments like massage therapy or body wraps can further stimulate circulation and lymphatic drainage, aiding in cellulite reduction. Consistency is key when combining treatments.

CHAPTER FIVE

MASSAGE TREATMENTS TO REDUCE CELLULITE

BENEFITS OF MASSAGE FOR REDUCING CELLULITE

In addition to increasing blood flow to the treated areas, massage also promotes the breakdown of fat deposits beneath the skin, further smoothing out cellulite. These are just a few of the many advantages of massage therapy for cellulite reduction. One of the main advantages is its ability to stimulate lymphatic drainage, which helps to remove toxins and excess fluid from the body's tissues. Over time, this process can reduce the appearance of cellulite dimples.

Regular massage therapy also improves skin elasticity and firmness by promoting the production of collagen, which not only helps reduce cellulite but also improves overall skin health and texture. Another important advantage of massage therapy is that it has the potential to reduce stress, which in turn can help reduce cellulite by balancing hormones like cortisol.

In conclusion, massage therapy can help reduce cellulite because it can improve blood circulation, stimulate lymphatic drainage, increase skin elasticity, and lower stress levels. These combined effects can eventually result in smoother skin texture and a decrease in the visible signs of cellulite.

VARIOUS MASSAGE TECHNIQUE TYPES

While many massage techniques target different aspects of tissue manipulation and circulation enhancement that are beneficial for cellulite reduction, one popular technique is deep tissue massage, which involves firm pressure applied to deeper layers of connective tissue and muscle to break down adhesions and knots that contribute to cellulite formation and promote smoother skin.

By gently stimulating lymphatic vessels, lymphatic drainage massage is an additional effective technique that reduces toxins and fluid retention in the body. It does this by encouraging the removal of waste products and excess fluid, which in turn reduces the appearance of cellulite dimples.

Furthermore, the connective tissue that envelops muscles and organs is stretched and released using myofascial release techniques. By releasing taut fascia, these treatments help enhance circulation and lessen the tension that accentuates the appearance of cellulite.

To summarize, various massage modalities, including deep tissue massage, lymphatic drainage massage, and myofascial release, target different aspects of tissue manipulation and circulation enhancement, which results in smoother skin texture and a reduced appearance of cellulite.

THE WAY THAT MASSAGE BOOSTS BLOOD CIRCULATION

The application of pressure to the skin and underlying tissues during a massage session dilates blood vessels, increasing blood flow to the treated areas. Better circulation aids in the removal of metabolic waste products and improves the delivery of oxygen and nutrients to cells, both of which are critical for the reduction of cellulite and overall health promotion.

Furthermore, massage promotes the breakdown of fat deposits that contribute to the formation of cellulite by stimulating the production of nitric oxide, a molecule that helps to relax blood vessels and improve blood flow.

By enhancing blood flow, massage improves the general health of skin tissues, promoting elasticity and minimizing the appearance of cellulite dimples.

To sum up, massage therapy enhances blood circulation through the dilation of blood vessels, the delivery of oxygen and nutrients to cells, and the assistance in eliminating metabolic waste products. These benefits are critical in the reduction of cellulite and maintenance of healthy skin tissue, ultimately leading to a more refined and firmer texture of the skin over time.

HOMEMADE MASSAGE TECHNIQUES

A cost-effective and convenient way to aid in the reduction of cellulite is to perform massage techniques at home. One such technique is dry brushing, which is a gentle circular motion that uses a natural bristle brush to gently brush the skin. This helps to exfoliate the skin, improve blood circulation, and stimulate lymphatic drainage—all of which are factors in the reduction of cellulite.

Using a cellulite massage tool, like a handheld roller or suction cup, is another do-it-yourself option. These tools are designed to apply mild pressure to specific areas, encouraging lymphatic drainage and breaking down fat deposits beneath the skin.

Regular use of these techniques can improve skin texture and minimize the appearance of cellulite dimples.

Furthermore, kneading, squeezing, and circular motions are some of the hand self-massage techniques that can help reduce cellulite. These techniques improve the appearance of cellulite over time by stimulating blood flow and lymphatic drainage.

It's important to use a moisturizing lotion or oil to minimize friction and maximize the benefits of these self-massage techniques.

In conclusion, self-massage, dry brushing, and cellulite massage tools are examples of do-it-yourself massage methods that can be used in conjunction with professional cellulite reduction treatments. These methods help to break down fat deposits beneath the skin's surface, improve blood circulation, and stimulate lymphatic drainage, which in turn promotes smoother skin texture and less cellulite dimples.

EXPERT MASSAGE SERVICES: WHAT TO ANTICIPATE

Through targeted techniques and expertise, professional massage services can significantly aid in cellulite reduction. One popular professional treatment is anti-cellulite massage, which combines techniques like deep tissue massage, lymphatic drainage, and myofascial release to effectively target cellulite-prone areas. These sessions are customized to meet the needs of each client and may require multiple sessions for best results.

Professional massage therapists use specific techniques to manipulate tissues, improve circulation, and stimulate lymphatic drainage, all of which help to reduce cellulite and improve skin tone. They will evaluate your skin condition and degree of cellulite to customize the treatment plan.

To further enhance the effects of massage on cellulite reduction, licensed massage therapists may also suggest complementary therapies like infrared therapy or body wraps. These therapies support overall skin health and texture by further detoxifying tissues, stimulating metabolism, and promoting the breakdown of fat deposits.

To summarize, customized treatment plans based on individual needs are provided by professional massage services for cellulite reduction. Techniques like deep tissue massage and lymphatic drainage are used to improve circulation, stimulate tissue detoxification, and gradually reduce cellulite dimples. These specialized treatments combine various techniques to effectively target cellulite-prone areas.

CHAPTER SIX

SUPPLEMENTAL DIETARY INTAKE AND CELLULITE

AN OVERVIEW OF SUPPLEMENTS TO REDUCE CELLULITE

Understanding the function and efficacy of supplements is crucial when looking into ways to reduce cellulite. Supplements typically make the following claims: they promote skin health, reduce cellulite appearance through different mechanisms, and contain common ingredients like vitamins, minerals, herbal extracts, and specially designed compounds that target cellulite.

These supplements are usually sold in different forms, like liquids, pills, capsules, or tablets, and each one claims to have a different effect on skin firmness and texture.

Understanding how these supplements work synergistically with a healthy diet and exercise regimen is key to maximizing their benefits.

Ingredients like collagen peptides, hyaluronic acid, and antioxidants like vitamins C and E are often highlighted for their potential to improve skin elasticity and reduce the dimpled appearance of cellulite. To start addressing cellulite with supplements, it's important to research and select products backed by scientific evidence and positive user reviews.

Supplements can help reduce cellulite, but they work best when paired with other lifestyle modifications like regular exercise, drinking plenty of water, and eating a balanced diet. Speaking with dermatologists or healthcare professionals can provide customized recommendations based on individual health conditions, ensuring safe and efficient supplementation for cellulite management.

MINERALS AND VITAMINS NEEDED FOR HEALTHY SKIN

Vitamin C, an antioxidant that promotes collagen production and helps maintain skin elasticity,

Vitamin E, a powerful antioxidant that shields skin cells from free radical damage and may eventually lessen the appearance of cellulite, and essential minerals like zinc and selenium, which support skin repair and renewal, are all important for maintaining skin health, which is essential for managing cellulite.

While dietary sources like fruits, vegetables, nuts, and seeds naturally contain these nutrients, supplements offer concentrated doses that may help target specific skin concerns like cellulite. Knowing the role of each vitamin and mineral in skin health empowers individuals to make informed choices when selecting supplements to support their cellulite reduction efforts. Including a variety of vitamins and minerals in your diet or supplementation plan can enhance skin resilience and reduce the visibility of cellulite.

To achieve safe and effective support for cellulite management, it is important to prioritize quality and potency when considering vitamin and mineral supplements for cellulite reduction. Look for supplements from reputable brands with transparent ingredient lists and third-party testing for purity and efficacy. Speaking with a healthcare provider or nutritionist can help tailor a supplement regimen that addresses specific skin needs and health goals.

THE EFFICIENCY OF HERBAL SUPPLEMENTS

Herbal supplements are a popular option for reducing cellulite because of their natural ingredients and perceived benefits. Ginkgo biloba, gotu kola, and horse chestnut extract are examples of ingredients that are frequently found in supplements that target cellulite because of their supposed benefits to promote collagen synthesis, improve circulation, and reduce inflammation. These herbs are also thought to support skin health by improving lymphatic drainage and blood flow, which may eventually reduce the appearance of cellulite.

Researching the efficacy and safety of herbal supplements is crucial when incorporating them into a cellulite reduction regimen.

Although some studies have shown promising results, individual factors such as skin type, lifestyle choices, and general health can affect the outcome of cellulite reduction. To maximize the potential benefits of herbal supplements, a holistic approach incorporating healthy diet choices, regular exercise, and adequate hydration is recommended.

By being aware of the mechanisms through which herbal supplements work to reduce cellulite, people can make well-informed decisions about how to incorporate them into their skincare routine. Speaking with a healthcare professional or herbalist can also offer helpful information about dosage, possible drug interactions, and reasonable expectations for smoother skin texture.

People can support their cellulite reduction goals and naturally promote overall skin health by incorporating herbal supplements responsibly and consistently.

WARNINGS AND THINGS TO THINK ABOUT

Supplements have the potential to help reduce cellulite, but it's important to use them carefully and thoughtfully. Not all supplements are regulated or proven to work, and some may worsen pre-existing medical conditions or interact with medications. Before beginning any supplement regimen for cellulite, people should do extensive research on products, paying particular attention to ingredients that are backed by credible scientific research and manufacturing standards.

Cellulite-targeting supplements may cause upset stomach, allergic reactions, or interactions with medications. It is important to carefully read product labels, adhere to recommended dosages, and monitor for any negative reactions while using these supplements.

A dermatologist or healthcare professional can offer specific advice on supplement safety, especially for those with underlying health issues or sensitivities.

Taking a proactive and informed approach to supplement use ensures safer and more effective results in managing cellulite over time. Supplements should be used in conjunction with a comprehensive approach to cellulite reduction that includes lifestyle modifications such as maintaining a healthy weight, exercising regularly, and staying hydrated. By combining supplements with these foundational practices, people can enhance their efforts to minimize cellulite appearance while supporting overall well-being.

TALKING WITH MEDICAL PROFESSIONALS

Healthcare providers can provide tailored guidance based on individual health history, current medications, and specific skin concerns, helping to tailor a supplement plan that aligns with overall wellness goals. This consultation allows for discussion of potential benefits, risks, and realistic expectations associated with supplement use for cellulite management.

Consulting with a healthcare provider is imperative before beginning any supplement regimen for cellulite reduction to ensure safety and efficacy.

In addition to providing targeted treatment approaches and supplements, healthcare providers can also perform assessments to identify underlying factors that contribute to the formation of cellulite, such as circulation issues or hormonal imbalances. By addressing these root causes, they can provide comprehensive care that supports long-term skin health and cellulite reduction.

A cellulite reduction strategy that incorporates recommendations from healthcare providers ensures a comprehensive approach that takes into account individual health needs and maximizes the effectiveness of supplements. Scheduling regular follow-up appointments enables individuals to monitor progress, make necessary adjustments to supplement regimens, and address any issues that may come up.

CHAPTER SEVEN

MEDICAL CELLULITE TREATMENTS

AN OVERVIEW OF THE AVAILABLE MEDICAL PROCEDURES

It's important to comprehend the range of procedures that are available when looking into medical treatments for cellulite reduction. These treatments are designed to reduce the appearance of cellulite by targeting underlying fat deposits and improving skin elasticity.

Some of the most popular procedures include injection therapies, liposuction, laser therapy, and mesotherapy. Each procedure has a different goal and method, but they all aim to improve skin texture and reduce the dimpled appearance that comes with cellulite.

A popular option because of its minimal discomfort and relatively short recovery time, laser therapy stands out as a non-invasive technique that uses focused laser energy to break down fat deposits and stimulate collagen production in the skin, helping to tighten the skin and reduce the visibility of cellulite over multiple sessions.

Injecting vitamins, enzymes, hormones, and plant extracts directly into the affected areas is known as mesotherapy or injection therapy. The goal of these injections is to break down fat cells and improve circulation, which can reduce cellulite and improve skin texture. Although mesotherapy is less popular than laser therapy, it offers targeted treatment and may be of interest to people seeking localized fat reduction with little downtime.

LASER THERAPY: ITS ADVANTAGES

Using cutting-edge technology, laser therapy targets fat cells located beneath the skin's surface. Deep tissue penetration of the laser energy breaks down fat deposits and promotes the production of collagen, which together smooth out the skin and gradually reduces the appearance of cellulite.

One of the main advantages of laser therapy is that it is non-invasive, which makes it a good option for people who are apprehensive about having surgery. Patients usually feel very little discomfort during the treatment, and any redness or swelling that occurs is usually temporary. Moreover, laser therapy sessions are usually brief, allowing patients to get back to their regular activities right away.

INJECTION THERAPIES AND MESOTHERAPY

By injecting specific formulations directly into the skin, mesotherapy, and injection therapies provide an additional method of reducing cellulite. These treatments consist of a series of injections that target fat cells and improve circulation, breaking down fat deposits, smoothing out cellulite, and improving skin firmness.

While mesotherapy can be effective in reducing cellulite, optimal results usually require multiple sessions spaced several weeks apart.

Patients may experience mild discomfort during the injections, along with possible bruising or swelling that resolves within a few days. The injections are applied precisely across the treatment area, ensuring even distribution of the active ingredients.

THE FUNCTION OF LIPOSUCTION IN REDUCING CELLULITE

Liposuction, a surgical technique that involves using tiny incisions to suction fat deposits from beneath the skin, is best known for its ability to remove fat, but it can also help reduce cellulite. Although liposuction targets deeper fat layers rather than cellulite directly, it can improve overall body contours and indirectly reduce the appearance of cellulite in treated areas.

Though liposuction is generally more invasive than non-surgical treatments and requires a longer recovery period, newer techniques such as laser-assisted liposuction or ultrasound-assisted liposuction may offer additional benefits for cellulite reduction.

These techniques help to tighten the skin and stimulate collagen production, which can enhance the smoothing effect on cellulite-prone areas.

SAFETY AND MEDICINAL TREATMENT CONSIDERATIONS

It's important to think about safety and potential risks before beginning any medical treatment for cellulite reduction. Although procedures like laser therapy and mesotherapy are generally safe when done by trained professionals, there is a chance of temporary discomfort, bruising, or infection at the injection sites.

To reduce this risk, patients should do their homework and select reputable clinics with experienced practitioners.

Finally, while medical treatments offer effective options for cellulite reduction, proper evaluation, and informed decision-making are crucial steps in ensuring a safe and successful outcome. Individuals with specific medical conditions or allergies should also speak with their healthcare provider before undergoing any cellulite treatment. It is important to understand realistic expectations and discuss treatment goals with a qualified specialist to achieve satisfactory results.

CHAPTER EIGHT

NATURAL THERAPIES AND AT-HOME REMEDIES

HOMEMADE CELLULITE TREATMENTS THAT WORK

DIY treatments can be a convenient and affordable option for those looking to reduce cellulite at home. One popular technique is dry brushing, which involves massaging the skin in circular motions with a natural bristle brush to improve circulation and lymphatic drainage, which gradually reduces the appearance of cellulite. Another effective method is coffee scrubbing, which involves rubbing coffee grounds mixed with a small amount of olive oil to tighten and reduce fluid retention in the skin.

Additionally, adding regular exercise to your routine can help reduce cellulite significantly. Exercises like cardio and strength training improve circulation and muscle tone, which can help smooth out the appearance of cellulite.

Eating a healthy diet high in fruits, vegetables, and lean proteins promotes skin health in general and reduces the buildup of toxins that cause cellulite formation.

THE VALUE OF DETOXIFICATION AND HYDRATION

Drinking enough water throughout the day can help flush out toxins from the body, improving skin elasticity and reducing the appearance of cellulite. You can also enhance the detoxifying properties of water by adding slices of cucumber or lemon. Herbal teas, such as dandelion or green tea, can also help with detoxification and promote healthier skin.

Dry sauna or steam room sessions are another good way to help the body get rid of toxins through sweat. This helps to improve circulation, which makes cellulite less noticeable. Eating foods high in antioxidants, like berries and leafy greens, regularly helps to support skin health and detoxification, which also helps to make skin look smoother.

ESSENTIAL OILS AND HERBAL REMEDIES

Natural methods of reducing cellulite include the use of herbal remedies and essential oils. For example, juniper oil, which has been shown to have detoxifying qualities, can be diluted with a carrier oil such as coconut oil and applied topically to improve circulation and decrease fluid retention.

Similarly, grapefruit essential oil has antioxidants that can break down fat cells and minimize the appearance of cellulite.

Gotu kola is another herbal remedy that works well; it can be applied topically as a cream or taken orally. It improves skin elasticity and reduces cellulite over time by increasing the production of collagen. You can also reduce cellulite from within by including herbs like cayenne pepper and ginger in your diet.

DIETARY CHANGES FOR NATURALLY REDUCED CELLULITE

Foods high in omega-3 fatty acids, like salmon and flaxseeds, support skin health and elasticity, minimizing the appearance of cellulite. Dietary changes are essential for natural cellulite reduction. Concentrate on consuming foods high in antioxidants, like berries, dark chocolate, and nuts, which help combat free radicals that contribute to cellulite formation.

Cutting back on salt is also a good idea because too much sodium causes fluid retention, which makes cellulite more visible. Instead, add flavor to your food with herbs and spices, which have the same effect as salt but don't harm your stomach.

Lean proteins and foods high in fiber also help you stay at a healthy weight and prevent fat from building up, which is another way to help reduce cellulite.

COMBINATION TREATMENTS FOR THE BEST OUTCOMES

Combining different therapies is often necessary to achieve the best results in cellulite reduction. For example, regular dry brushing sessions combined with a healthy diet and plenty of water improve circulation and aid in the removal of toxins, which in turn causes cellulite to gradually disappear. Strength training exercises combined with herbal remedies and essential oils can further tone muscles and improve the texture of the skin.

Additionally, in addition to home remedies, professional treatments like radiofrequency therapy or lymphatic drainage massage can target deeper layers of cellulite and promote collagen production; these therapies, when paired with lifestyle modifications like consistent exercise and a balanced diet, can maximize results and improve the overall appearance of skin; incorporating these approaches into a holistic cellulite reduction regimen guarantees comprehensive care and long-lasting results.

CHAPTER NINE

SUSTAINING OUTCOMES AND AVOIDING CELLULITE

TECHNIQUES FOR PREVENTING CELLULITE OVER TIME

A comprehensive strategy that addresses lifestyle choices, as well as targeted treatments, is necessary for long-term cellulite prevention. Eating a balanced diet high in fruits, vegetables, and lean proteins while reducing sugar and processed food intake helps maintain a healthy weight and prevents the buildup of fat that contributes to cellulite. Regular exercise, including cardiovascular and strength training, improves circulation and tones muscles, which gradually reduces the appearance of cellulite. Hydration is also essential, as it helps eliminate toxins from the body and keeps the skin hydrated and supple.

Apart from diet and exercise, using massage or dry brushing techniques can help break down fat deposits under the skin and stimulate lymphatic drainage; these methods also improve circulation and collagen production, which results in smoother skin texture; using cellulite creams or lotions with ingredients like retinol or caffeine can temporarily tighten the skin and lessen the appearance of cellulite; and finally, sticking to a regular regimen of these preventive measures is crucial for long-term success in managing cellulite.

THE VALUE OF TREATMENT CONSISTENCY

Maintaining a regular schedule when implementing a treatment plan, whether it involves dietary modifications, exercise regimens, or skincare routines, ensures that the body adapts and responds positively to the interventions. For example, following a daily routine of dry brushing or massaging affected areas helps improve blood circulation and lymphatic drainage, which are critical in reducing cellulite visibility. Consistency is crucial in cellulite reduction treatments because it allows the cumulative effects of dietary changes, exercise routines, and topical treatments to take full effect.

When it comes to diet, following a well-balanced and health-promoting diet helps manage weight and reduce the underlying factors that contribute to the formation of cellulite. Exercise, on the other hand, tones muscles and burns fat, making areas of the body more likely to appear cellulite-free. Finally, when it comes to cellulite creams or serums, using them as prescribed helps the active ingredients to work their way into the skin and maximize their effectiveness over time.

All things considered, the benefit of consistency is that it can promote slow but steady improvements in the reduction of cellulite. People who incorporate treatments into their daily or weekly routine and follow through on them can maximize their efforts in the long run to attain skin that is smoother and looks healthier.

HOW TO KEEP AN EYE ON AND TRACK DEVELOPMENT

Taking regular photos of the areas being treated under consistent lighting conditions and angles is an effective way to keep track of progress and assess the effectiveness of treatments.

Comparing these photos over time provides a visual representation of changes in cellulite visibility, which offers motivation and insight into the effectiveness of the chosen treatments.

Moreover, measuring body circumferences or using body fat calipers can provide quantitative data on changes in body composition and cellulite severity. Keeping a journal or diary is another way to track progress, as it allows individuals to record their daily or weekly activities related to cellulite reduction, such as dietary changes, exercise routines, and skincare regimens. This helps track adherence to the treatment plan and allows for adjustments based on observed outcomes.

A systematic approach to monitoring and tracking progress can help individuals make informed decisions about their cellulite reduction strategies and maintain motivation throughout their journey. Subjective assessments, such as self-perceived improvements in skin texture or firmness, can also be included to monitor progress. These self-evaluations can be supplemented by professional evaluations, such as consultations with dermatologists or aestheticians, who can provide expert advice and objective measurements of cellulite severity.

CHANGING TREATMENTS IN RESPONSE TO OUTCOMES

To maximize cellulite reduction efforts and achieve desired results, it is imperative to make adjustments to treatments based on observed results. If, after a reasonable period, initial treatments do not produce noticeable improvements, it may be necessary to reassess and modify the approach. This may entail speaking with a healthcare professional or skincare expert to discuss other options or to modify existing treatments to better suit specific needs and skin types.

For example, if a specific cellulite cream or lotion is not working well, trying other products with different active ingredients or formulations might be helpful. You could also try varying the amount of pressure or frequency that you massage or use dries brushing techniques to improve their ability to increase circulation and decrease the appearance of cellulite. Finally, if lifestyle factors like exercise and diet are important, making changes to these under professional guidance can eventually improve results.

Individuals can customize their cellulite reduction strategies to achieve optimal results effectively and sustainably by being flexible and open to trying new approaches. Regularly reviewing progress through objective measures like photographs or body measurements helps in identifying when adjustments are needed.

CREATING WELL-BEING ROUTINES FOR LONG-TERM SUCCESS

Developing healthy habits is essential to maintaining cellulite reduction results over time. This entails incorporating lifestyle adjustments that support overall body composition and skin health. For example, a balanced diet high in antioxidants, vitamins, and minerals stimulates collagen production and skin elasticity in addition to reducing cellulite. Lean proteins and healthy fats also support muscle tone and decrease fat accumulation, which contributes to smoother skin texture.

Frequent exercise is still important because it improves blood flow, builds muscle, and burns fat. Adding cardiovascular and strength training to your weekly routine helps target areas of your body that are prone to cellulite and improves overall body contour. Staying hydrated is also important because it helps to flush out toxins and keeps your skin hydrated, which keeps it supple and helps to reduce the appearance of cellulite.

Together with these basic practices, stress-reduction methods like yoga, meditation, or deep breathing exercises support skin health by lowering cortisol levels, which can contribute to the development of cellulite. Getting enough sleep each night enables the body to repair and regenerate, promoting healthier skin and body function. People who regularly prioritize these healthy habits can maintain their efforts to reduce cellulite and experience long-lasting improvements in their overall appearance and well-being.

CHAPTER TEN
FAQS & FREQUENTLY ASKED QUESTIONS
TAKING CARE OF SAFETY ISSUES

Before beginning any treatment, speak with a qualified healthcare provider to determine your suitability and address any underlying health concerns. They can offer you personalized advice based on your medical history and current state of health. You should also look up the credentials of the practitioner or clinic offering the treatments to make sure they are qualified and experienced in cellulite reduction procedures. Safety should always come first when starting any kind of treatment for cellulite reduction.

Prioritizing safety from the beginning allows you to undergo cellulite reduction procedures with confidence and peace of mind. Common safety concerns include allergic reactions to treatment ingredients, skin sensitivity, or adverse reactions to equipment used during procedures. By discussing these factors with your healthcare provider, you can make an informed decision about which treatments are safest for you. It's also important to carefully follow post-treatment care instructions to minimize risks and optimize results.

CONTROLLING ANTICIPATIONS FOR CELLULITE THERAPY

While cellulite reduction treatments can improve the appearance of cellulite, they may not eliminate it. It is important to manage expectations when considering cellulite reduction treatments because the results can vary depending on individual factors like skin type, severity of cellulite, and overall health. You should discuss realistic goals with your healthcare provider and be aware that multiple sessions may be required to achieve optimal results.

A timeline for when to expect visible changes can be provided by your healthcare provider, who may also recommend complementary therapies or lifestyle changes to enhance results. Most cellulite reduction treatments require patience, as results usually develop gradually over weeks to months. It's important to maintain realistic expectations about the extent of improvement you can achieve. Keeping a positive but realistic mindset throughout your treatment journey will help you better appreciate and celebrate the progress made.

SETTING UP A BUDGET TO REDUCE CELLULITE

Pricing for cellulite reduction treatments can vary greatly depending on the type of procedure, the location of the clinic, and the number of sessions required. Research different providers to compare costs and take into account any financing options or package deals that may offer savings. When creating a budget for cellulite reduction, it is important to account for both the cost of treatments and any additional expenses such as consultations, follow-up visits, and skin care products recommended for maintenance.

Prioritize treatments that fit within your budget without sacrificing quality or safety. Knowing the full financial commitment involved in cellulite reduction treatments can help you plan effectively and avoid unforeseen costs along the way. Budgeting should also include potential expenses for aftercare products or supplements recommended by your healthcare provider.

HANDLING SIDE EFFECTS OF TREATMENT

It's important to discuss potential side effects with your healthcare provider before starting treatment so you can be prepared and know what to expect. Like any cosmetic procedure, cellulite reduction treatments can have side effects, which vary depending on the type of treatment and individual skin sensitivity. Common side effects may include temporary redness, bruising, swelling, or mild discomfort at the treatment site.

To minimize side effects and maximize results, carefully follow your provider's post-treatment instructions. These may include using cold compresses or soothing creams to reduce swelling and discomfort. You should also avoid sun exposure and strenuous exercise right after treatment. If you experience any unexpected or severe side effects, get in touch with your healthcare provider for advice and reassurance.

MODIFICATIONS TO YOUR LIFESTYLE FOR CONTINUOUS IMPROVEMENT

Incorporating regular exercise, such as strength training and cardio, can help improve circulation and tone muscles, which may contribute to reducing the appearance of cellulite. Eating a balanced diet rich in fruits, vegetables, lean proteins, and healthy fats can also support skin elasticity and overall skin health. Long-term results from cellulite reduction treatments often require lifestyle adjustments to support skin health and overall well-being.

Avoiding smoking and excessive alcohol consumption can also benefit skin health and improve treatment outcomes. Lastly, stress management techniques like yoga, meditation, or deep breathing exercises can reduce cortisol levels, which can contribute to cellulite formation. By making these lifestyle adjustments, you can support the results of cellulite reduction treatments and promote overall skin wellness. Drinking plenty of water throughout the day is essential for maintaining skin elasticity and reducing the appearance of cellulite.